YOUR KNOWLEDGE HAS VALUE

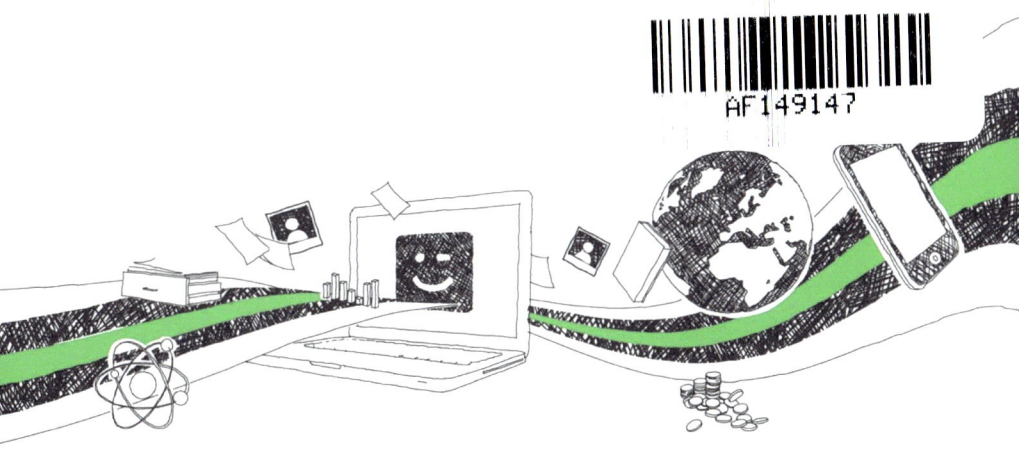

TariQual Islam Sajeeb

Hormonal effect on MRI

GRIN Verlag

Bibliografische Information der Deutschen Nationalbibliothek:

Die Deutsche Bibliothek verzeichnet diese Publikation in der Deutschen National-
bibliografie; detaillierte bibliografische Daten sind im Internet über http://dnb.d-
nb.de/ abrufbar.

Imprint:

Copyright © 2013 GRIN Verlag GmbH
Druck und Bindung: Books on Demand GmbH, Norderstedt Germany
ISBN: 978-3-656-64421-7

This book at GRIN:

http://www.grin.com/en/e-book/272336/hormonal-effect-on-mri

GRIN - Your knowledge has value

Der GRIN Verlag publiziert seit 1998 wissenschaftliche Arbeiten von Studenten, Hochschullehrern und anderen Akademikern als eBook und gedrucktes Buch. Die Verlagswebsite www.grin.com ist die ideale Plattform zur Veröffentlichung von Hausarbeiten, Abschlussarbeiten, wissenschaftlichen Aufsätzen, Dissertationen und Fachbüchern.

Visit us on the internet:

http://www.grin.com/

http://www.facebook.com/grincom

http://www.twitter.com/grin_com

Hormonal Effect on MRI

Introduction

At the age of 8-13years all the women faces some sort of changes in her life. Starting of menstruation, change in the body and mind (Ghai, 2012). Hormonal changes stimulates this changes in them (Hall, 2010). This hormonal change stimulates various changes in their body. One of the changes is the development of breast (Hall, 2010). The breast is a body part, which differ in size and function in male and female. The female breast is containing mammary gland which produces milk to feed infant (Boron & Boulpaep, 2012). Both men and women develop their breast from same embryological tissues (Hall, 2010). In puberty different hormones especially estrogen works in breast development (Russo & Russo, 2008). On the other hand male hormone testosterone doesn't have this function.

Hormonal influences on breast tissue during the normal menstrual cycle and importance on MRI

Menstruation cycle is an essential part for female. It is the changes in the uterus and ovary to reproduction of sexuality (Sherwood, 2010; Silverthorn, Johnson, & Ober, 2007). It is very essential for maturation of the women ovum and preparing the uterus for pregnancy. This cycle only occurs in fertile female humans (Hall, 2010; Silverthorn, et al., 2007). In the menstrual cycle there are many hormonal changes occurs in female body. The menstrual cycle occurs in two phases- the follicular phase or proliferative phase and the luteal or ovulatory phase(Hall, 2010).

In the menstrual cycle many hormonal changes occur. Three two main hormones which effects significantly in menstrual cycle. The estrogen is a hormone which gives the feeling of good. It gives energy with the help of testosterone and increase sex drive. Increased level of estrogen makes a women more feminine (Ghai, 2012). Progesterone is a tranquilizing hormone. It slows down the body a little. Increased level of progesterone lead to depression (Ghai, 2012). At the time of this cycle estrogen and progesterone stimulate the breasts to prepare for possible fertilization (Hall, 2010). The figure-1 shows the different hormonal changes according to days. This figure has adapted from(Rosenblatt, 2007)

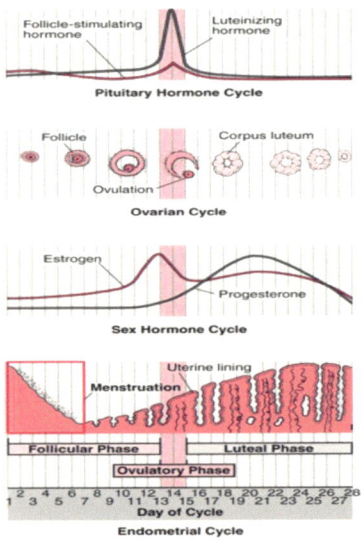

Figure:1 Phases of menstrual cycle adapted from(Rosenblatt, 2007).

Premenopausal ladies aged 40–49 years, there was a tiny low however statistically important variation in breast density by time within the cycle. Having a mammogram throughout the cyst part reduced the probability of breast density being classified as "extremely dense" as compared with having a mammogram throughout the stage (Ellis, 2009). This association (decreased breast density within the cyst part of the catamenial cycle) was stronger for ladies whose body mass index was capable or under the median, a gaggle that's rather more doubtless to be characterized as having very dense breasts, than for ladies whose body mass index was on top of the median(White.E.et.al, 1998).

It is biologically plausible that mammographic breast density, that could be a live of the proportion of the breast occupied by connective and animal tissue, would vary by time within the cycle as results of the results of variation within the levels of current hormones. Proof suggests that accrued secretion levels are related to accrued breast density(White.E.et.al, 1998). Studies of breast changes at the cellular level have shown that proliferation will increase 2-3 fold within the endocrine vs. follicular phase of the cycle. Thus, the rise in MRI FGT% we have a tendency to determine within the phase could also be reflective of exaggerated proliferation. However, is that cycle part was calculable supported self-report of cycle length, which cannot be used to dependably distinguish ovulatory vs. non-ovulatory cycles or temporal order of cycle phases as a result of the substantial variability between- and within-women in discharge cycle characteristics (Clendenen et al., 2012). It absolutely was determined increasing imaging FGT% and higher ADC and T2 in FGT within the endocrine vs. cyst part of the cycle, suggesting that FGT%, ADC, and T2 could also be of interest in future imaging studies examining the consequences of secretion exposures on the breast tissue. There's no pattern of breast tissue changes throughout the OC cycle (Clendenen, et al., 2012).

What are BRCA 1 and BRCA 2 genes? Implications for a patient who has a harmful BRCA gene mutation, and how are such patients managed clinically

BRCA1 and BRCA2 are genes in human body which produces tumor suppressor proteins. This type of proteins repairs damaged DNA and also helps to ensuring in the stability of the genetic materials of the cells .If these genes mutated or if the functions of these proteins doesn't remain functioning correctly then DNA damage may not be repaired correctly (Campeau, Foulkes, & Tischkowitz, 2008). As a result abnormal cell growth will be occurring this may lead to cancer. Some specific inherited mutations in these genes increase the risk of breast cancer. This is also associated with the increased risk of many other type of cancer (Campeau, et al., 2008). Mutation of BRCA1 and BRCA2 is the cause of 20-25% of breast cancer. Breast cancers for this reason are usually developed in the younger age. Mutation of BRCA1 and BRCA2 can be genetically gained from a person's mother or father. If a parent is carrying a mutation of these genes has 50% more vulnerability for gaining this mutation (Bolton et al., 2012).

To manage this type of patient we need to go through several steps. There are various screening options and interventions are available to manage BRCA-related cancer risks.

Screening

An intensive cancer screening program is sometimes suggested for ladies with harmful or suspected harmful BRCA mutations so as to find new cancers as early as doable. A typical recommendation includes frequent carcinoma screening yet as tests to find sex gland cancer. Breast imaging studies typically embody a breast imaging (magnetic resonance imaging) once a year, starting between ages twenty and thirty, looking on the age at that any relatives were diagnosed with carcinoma (Morris & Gordon, 2010). Mammograms square measure generally used solely at advanced age as there's reason to believe that BRCA carriers square measure additional vulnerable to carcinoma induction by X-ray harm than general population (Morris & Gordon, 2010). Breast imaging studies typically embody a breast imaging (magnetic resonance imaging) once a year, starting between ages twenty and thirty, looking on the age at that any relatives were diagnosed with carcinoma. Mammograms square measure generally used solely at advanced age as there's reason to believe that BRCA carriers square measure additional vulnerable to carcinoma induction by X-ray harm than general population (Morris & Gordon, 2010). Alternatives embody breast imaging, CT scans, PET scans, scintimammography, elastography, diagnostic procedure, ductal irrigation, and experimental screening protocols, a number of that hope to spot biomarkers for carcinoma (molecules that seem within the blood once carcinoma begins (Morris & Gordon, 2010).

Prophylactic mastectomy

In a lady who has not developed carcinoma, removing the breasts could cut back her risk of ever being diagnosed with carcinoma by ninetieth, to level that's some 0.5 the common woman's risk. Bilateral ablation is that the removal of each breast by a breast operating surgeon. The changed mastectomy is merely employed in girls diagnosed with invasive carcinoma. Techniques for prophylactic mastectomies include(Morris & Gordon, 2010):

- ❖ Simple ablation, which is usually recommended for ladies not having breast reconstruction, leaves quantity} amount of breast tissue within the body and thus achieves the best risk reduction. Additionally to prophylactic use, it's additionally employed by girls UN agencies are diagnosed with earlier stages of cancer(Morris & Gordon, 2010).
- ❖ Skin-sparing ablation removes the tissue of the breast, nipple, and areola, however leave the "excess" skin in situ for reconstruction. it's less visible connective tissue than an easy ablation(Morris & Gordon, 2010).
- ❖ Nipple-sparing ablation removes the breast tissue, however leaves the mamilla and also the areola intact for an additional natural look(Morris & Gordon, 2010).
- ❖ Subcutaneous ablation removes the breast tissue, however leaves the mamilla and areola intact. The scars area unit hidden within the inframammary fold below the breast(Morris & Gordon, 2010).
- ❖ Areola-sparing ablation removes the breast tissue and also the mamilla, however not the areola(Morris & Gordon, 2010).
- ❖ Nerve-sparing ablation is a shot to keep up the nerves that offer sensation to the heal the breasts. Breasts that have undergone any of those surgeries have a lot of less perception than natural breasts. Nerve-sparing techniques area unit a shot to retain some feeling within the breasts, with restricted and infrequently solely partial success(Morris & Gordon, 2010).

Intra-capsular and Extra-capsular rupture and their MRI appearances

An implant rupture may be a recognized complication of an implant. It will be intra or additional capsular. An intra-capsular rupture happens once the shell of the implant ruptures however the fibrous capsule shaped by the breast remains intact. Polymer doesn't freely extravasate. This makes it tough to notice on clinical test or diagnostic technique. Intra-capsular rupture is best seen on tomography.

An extra-capsular rupture will result in a modification within the implant contour and should be detected on clinical examination or diagnostic technique. Associate degree extra-capsular rupture implies intra-capsular rupture additionally.

Radiographic options

General

In associate degree intra-capsular rupture the contents of the implant ar contained by the fibrous scar, whereas the shell seems as a bunch of wavy lines. This has been termed the "linguine sign" and has been most ordinarily delineated with adult male imaging. The "keyhole sign, noose sign or teardrop sign" is that the look of polymer on each side of a radial fold associate degreed conjointly suggests an implant rupture (O'Brien, 2009)

Breast MRI

Considered most sensitive for detection of implant rupture. Typically doesn't needed distinction if the indication is entirely for this purpose. Non-contrast tomography may additionally be able to distinguish between polymer and / or saline implants by mistreatment polymer or water solely sequences. With the utilization of multi-planar imaging, adult male may additionally be able to distinguish between radial folds or true ruptures (O'Brien, 2009). A 'linguine sign' could also be seen that is restricted for associate degree intra-capsular rupture is because of the free floating shell among the implant (Clendenen, et al., 2012). A gross extra-capsular rupture is obvious as free polymer, cut loose the implant, which has extended on the far side the implant capsule into the breast or cavity. Free polymer has associate degree inflated signal in T2-stir weighted sequence with none sweetening in T1 weighted fat-suppressed sequence(O'Brien, 2009).

The "salad oil sign" has conjointly been delineated during a double lumen implant rupture, wherever there's mixture of the saline and polymer, though this on its own is non-specific (Clendenen, et al., 2012).

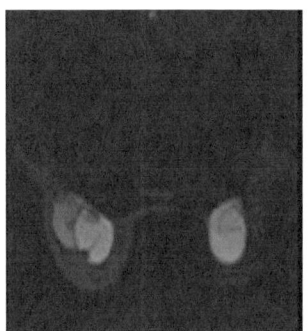 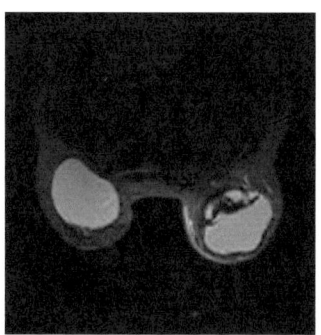

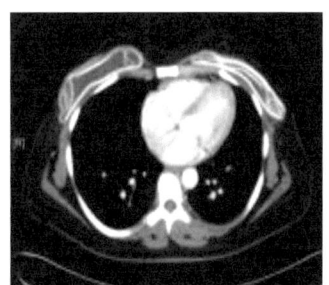 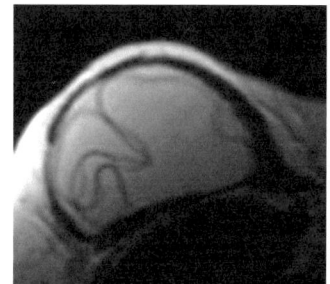

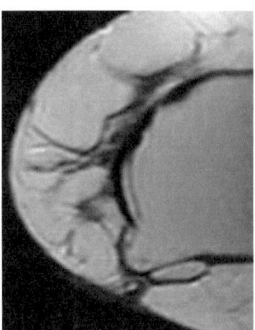

MRI Images of intra-capsular and extra-capsular rupture

References

1. Bolton, K. L., Chenevix-Trench, G., Goh, C., Sadetzki, S., Ramus, S. J., Karlan, B. Y., . . . McGuffog, L. (2012). Association between BRCA1 and BRCA2 mutations and survival in women with invasive epithelial ovarian cancer. *JAMA: the journal of the American Medical Association, 307*(4), 382-389.

2. Boron, W. F., & Boulpaep, E. L. (2012). *Medical Physiology, 2e Updated Edition: with STUDENT CONSULT Online Access*: Elsevier Health Sciences.

3. Campeau, P. M., Foulkes, W. D., & Tischkowitz, M. D. (2008). Hereditary breast cancer: new genetic developments, new therapeutic avenues. *Human genetics, 124*(1), 31-42.

4. Clendenen, T. V., Kim, S., Moy, L., Wan, L., Rusinek, H., Stanczyk, F. Z., . . . Zeleniuch-Jacquotte, A. (2012). Magnetic resonance imaging (MRI) of hormone-induced breast changes in young premenopausal women. *Magnetic Resonance Imaging*.

5. Ellis, R. L. (2009). Optimal timing of breast MRI examinations for premenopausal women who do not have a normal menstrual cycle. *American Journal of Roentgenology, 193*(6), 1738-1740.

6. Ghai, C. (2012). *A textbook of practical physiology*: Jaypee Brothers Medical Pub.

7. Hall, J. E. (2010). *Guyton and Hall Textbook of Medical Physiology: Enhanced E-book*: Elsevier Health Sciences.

8. Morris, J. L., & Gordon, O. K. (2010). *Positive Results: Making the Best Decisions when You're at High Risk for Breast Or Ovarian Cancer*: Prometheus Books.

9. O'Brien, W. (2009). *Top 3 differentials in radiology: a case review*: Thieme.

10. Rosenblatt, P. L. (Producer). (2007, July). Menstrual Cycle. *The Merck manual*. Retrieved from http://www.merckmanuals.com/home/womens_health_issues/biology_of_the_female_rep roductive_system/menstrual_cycle.html

11. Russo, J., & Russo, I. H. (2008). Breast development, hormones and cancer *Innovative Endocrinology of Cancer* (pp. 52-56): Springer.

12. Sherwood, L. (2010). *Fundamentals of Human Physiology*: Cengage Learning.

13. Silverthorn, D. U., Johnson, B. R., & Ober, W. C. (2007). *Human physiology*: Pearson/Benjamin Cummings.

14. White.E.et.al. (1998). Variation in Mammographic Breast Density by Time in Menstrual Cycle Among Women Aged 40–49 Years. *JNCI J Natl Cancer Inst*, Pp. 906-910.